One, seven, three, five—
Nothing to rely on in this or
     any world;
Nighttime falls and the water is
     flooded with moonlight.
Here in the Dragon's jaws:
Many exquisite jewels.
—the eleventh-century Zen
     master and poet Setcho
     Juken

How to Be Sick

Your Pocket Companion

Toni Bernhard

Wisdom

Wisdom Publications
199 Elm Street
Somerville, MA 02144 USA
wisdomexperience.org

Library of Congress Cataloging-in-Publication Data
Names: Bernhard, Toni, author.
Title: How to be sick: your pocket companion / Toni Bernhard.
Description: Somerville, MA, USA: Wisdom Publications, 2020.
Identifiers: LCCN 2019049778 (print) | LCCN 2019049779 (ebook) |
    ISBN 9781614296768 (pbk: acid-free paper) | ISBN 9781614296775 (ebook)
Subjects: LCSH: Religious life—Buddhism. | Chronically ill—Religious life.
    | Caregivers—Religious life. | Chronic diseases—Religious aspects—
    Buddhism.
Classification: LCC BQ5400 .B46 2020 (print) | LCC BQ5400 (ebook) |
    DDC 294.3/4442—dc23
LC record available at https://lccn.loc.gov/2019049778
LC ebook record available at https://lccn.loc.gov/2019049779

ISBN 978-1-61429-676-8 ebook ISBN 978-1-61429-677-5

24 23 22 21 20   5 4 3 2 1

Cover design by Phil Pascuzzo. Interior design by Tony Lulek.

Praise for *How to Be Sick:*
A Buddhist-Inspired Guide for the
Chronically Ill and Their Caregivers

"This book can bring you more fully alive by healing your spirit."
—Tara Brach, author of *Radical Acceptance*

"Beautiful, heartfelt, and immensely courageous. Truly worth reading."
—Sharon Salzberg, author of *Lovingkindness*

"This is a book for all of us."
—Sylvia Boorstein, author of *Happiness Is an Inside Job*

"Practical, wise, and full of heart."
—James Baraz, author of *Awakening Joy*

"Told with relentless honesty and clarity."
—Stephen Batchelor, author of *Confession of a Buddhist Atheist*

Introduction

I created this edition of *How to Be Sick* in response to requests for a smaller, pocket-sized version: something that people can carry with them and refer to when obstacles arise in their day—as obstacles inevitably do.

In 2001, I fell ill with what appeared to be an acute viral infection, but I never recovered. I'm mostly housebound, often bedbound with the aches and pains and lack of stamina that characterize the flu.

For years, I blamed myself for becoming chronically ill, as if I lacked the strength of character to recover my health. Gradually, and with the help of the Buddha's down-to-earth teachings, I realized that everyone's life is a mixture of pleasant and unpleasant experiences. Chronic illness is one of those unpleasant experiences; it's a presence in my life every day, but it doesn't touch the heart of who I am.

You can't always choose the challenges you'll have to face in life, but you can learn not to let those challenges diminish you. Finding a measure of peace and happiness depends not on the state of your health but on how you respond to it. If you respond with bitterness and anger, you become a bitter and angry person, and that adds a layer of mental suffering to the difficulties you're already facing. Mental suffering can take two forms: painful emotions—frustration, anger, worry, fear (sometimes all at the same time!)—and irrational and stressful thinking patterns that trap you in their loops, such as talking yourself into believing you'll never enjoy yourself again or that family and friends don't care about you anymore.

This book is a handy reference guide that offers strategies and practices to alleviate such mental suffering. It's organized by the challenges that the chronically ill and their caregivers face. (Chronic illness includes chronic pain and can include mental illness, such as depression and PTSD.) You can read it front to back, or you can look up the challenges you're facing at the moment and read through my recommendations. You'll notice some repetition in the book; this is because some of my suggestions, such as Three-Breath Practice, are useful in a variety of situations. If a strategy or practice doesn't resonate with you, that's fine; move on to the next one.

With chronic illness as your starting point, I hope you'll use this book to heal your mind and build a new and fulfilling life.

The Challenges

THE CHALLENGE
Not Engaging in Self-Blame

I know from experience that nothing positive comes from directing blame at yourself. Anybody can get sick, physically or mentally, and anybody can develop chronic pain. It can happen when you're young. It can happen when you're older.

Sadly, self-blame is often the habitual response when you're faced with one of the challenges that are the subjects of this book. A treatment didn't work? Somehow, it's your fault. You received dismissive care from a doctor? Somehow, you did something wrong at the appointment.

Blaming yourself for something that isn't your fault wastes your precious energy. Instead, spend your time doing what you can to ease your symptoms and to build the best life you can for yourself.

The suggestions and practices that follow will help put an end to the blame game.

Recognize that a lack of control over much that happens to you is an inescapable reality of the human condition.

If you had control over what happened to you, you'd order up a lifetime of perfect health. I certainly would. But life doesn't work that way. At some point, all of us must grapple with health challenges that are beyond our ability to control.

You are not alone in this. This is simply how and when it happened to you.

No blame!

*Use Three-Breath Practice to shift your
attention from self-blame to what's
happening in your immediate experience.*

This mindfulness practice is easy but powerful. All you need do is *pause*—and bring your
full attention to the physical sensation of three
consecutive in-breaths and out-breaths.

Because the sensations of the breath
always occur in the present moment, this
practice puts you in the present moment.
This prevents you from remaining lost in self-
judgmental thoughts.

Three-Breath Practice can be done any
time, any place, and in any posture. Your eyes
can be opened or closed.

The more you practice it, the earlier you'll
begin noticing that a judgmental thought has
arisen. Catching it early like this can keep it
from escalating into full-blown self-blame.

*Be sure that embarrassment isn't
contributing to your self-blame.*

Embarrassment is the painful, self-conscious feeling that you're violating a social norm because you can't regain your health. It arises as a result of childhood and cultural conditioning that cause you to hold yourself to unrealistically high standards; when you can't meet them, you feel embarrassed, even ashamed.

The unrealistic standard at work here is that perfect health is within your power if you'd just eat right, exercise, etc. This distorted view is fueled by the media and often by the people right around you.

To overcome embarrassment, first, recognize that its source is unrealistic expectations, and then remind yourself that pain and illness come with the human experience. You don't control when they'll show up or how long they'll stick around. There's nothing to feel embarrassed about.

Think of words that address the pain of self-
blame, and recite them to yourself
in a kind and soothing manner.

Consider this from Pema Chödrön, a teacher of Tibetan Buddhism: "The most difficult times for many of us are those we give ourselves."

If you are your own harshest critic, you can find relief from that emotional suffering by coming up with words that capture how painful it is to engage in self-blame. Then gently repeat them to yourself. Your words might be similar to these: "Blaming myself for something that isn't under my control hurts as if it's a self-inflicted wound" or "It's upsetting to realize that I treat myself more harshly than I'd ever treat others; that's not fair to me."

Expressing understanding and compassion for yourself in this way disarms self-blame. You are, in effect, taking away its power over you. As a result, it might just make a hasty exit!

"Count each separate day as a separate life" (as advised by the Roman philosopher Seneca).

Try counting each *moment* as a separate life, too. You may have blamed yourself for being chronically ill in the last moment, but this is a new moment—a new life.

In this new life, instead of criticizing yourself for something that's not your fault, treat yourself with understanding and compassion.

And if you fall back into your old habit of self-blame, it's okay because, in the next moment, you can start anew!

THE CHALLENGE
Making Peace with Your Inability to Know What the Future Holds for You

We'd all like certainty in our lives. If you're like me, the desire to know what's going to happen to you would sit near the top of your wish list. But none of us can know.

One of the conditions of being alive is that you're subject to constant change and all it implies, including uncertainty, unpredictability, and a lack of control over much that happens to you.

Being chronically ill can make all of life feel problematic, from what social commitments to make to whether you'll be able to handle an emergency.

Here are some strategies and practices to help you find a measure of peace and contentment in the midst of life's uncertainty.

Use Three-Breath Practice to bring your attention to your present-moment experience, instead of dwelling on a future you can't possibly know.

When you become aware that you're lost in worrisome thoughts about the future, *pause*, and switch your attention to the physical sensation of three in-breaths and three out-breaths in a row. Take your time.

Three-Breath Practice offers relief from distressing thoughts and emotions because it shifts your attention to what's going on in your immediate experience.

It also helps you find things to enjoy that are available to you right now. Repeat as necessary!

When thoughts about the future give rise to anxiety or other painful emotions, turn to self-compassion to ease your suffering.

The way you treat yourself is one of the few things you control in life. There's no reason to be anything but kind to yourself, both in your speech and your actions. Compassion-ate action includes taking care of your needs and looking for ways to enjoy yourself despite your limitations.

To engage in compassionate self-talk, think of words that speak directly to how hard it is to long for certainty in an uncer-tain world. Then recite them to yourself in a soothing voice, words such as "It's scary not to know what the future holds for me" or "My ongoing worry about the future is so emotionally draining."

When you give voice to your feelings in this way, you're letting yourself know that you care about your suffering. This alone will ease your emotional pain.

Keep a Don't-Know Mind about the future.

You don't know what the future holds for you, long-term. You don't even know for sure what tomorrow will bring.

The Korean Zen master Seung Sahn's instruction to keep a Don't-Know Mind is an invitation to lay down the burden of constantly striving to know the unknowable.

It's remarkably liberating to be able to say, "I don't know." Those words free you to let your life unfold as it may without the futile effort on your part to control everything.

Keeping a Don't-Know Mind is also an invaluable way to stop yourself from believing distressing assumptions, such as "The future holds only pain and heartbreak for me." You can't know this. Better days may be just around the corner. Keep your heart and mind open to all possibilities.

*Cultivate equanimity to alleviate any fear or
other painful emotions that are present when
you think about the future.*

Equanimity is characterized by an even-
tempered contentment that arises when you
feel okay about your life even though you
don't know what the future has in store.

A student once asked the spiritual teacher
Jiddu Krishnamurti what his secret to peace
and contentment was. He leaned over and
whispered to the student: "I don't mind what
happens."

To cultivate equanimity in this way, start
by gently acknowledging any worry or fear
you're experiencing at the moment. Then try
to imagine what it would be like to not mind
what was going to happen next in your life.

This can be a challenge, so if it was too
hard to imagine, wait a bit and try again.

THE CHALLENGE
Responding Skillfully to the Relentlessness of Symptoms

If you're like me, you've had days when your symptoms made you cry out, "Enough is enough. *Get out of here!*"

Although saying this may temporarily feel good, it's *not* good for your symptoms to treat them as the enemy. It can even intensify them because emotions such as anger are felt in the body. Anger and other painful emotions drain your energy, and can also lead to tightening of muscles, digestive disturbances, and sleep disruption.

When you're upset and angry about the relentlessness of your symptoms, I hope the suggestions and practices that follow will help you heal emotionally.

Recognize that the symptoms of chronic illness are as changeable as the weather.

Even though you're feeling overwhelmed by your symptoms at the moment, don't forget that they're in constant flux, just like the weather.

Consider this poem from the thirteenth-century Zen master Eihei Dogen:

Without the bitterest cold that
   penetrates to the very bone,
How can plum blossoms send
   forth their fragrance all over
   the universe?

Without trying to force any sadness to go away, let his words encourage you to patiently wait until the bitter cold of your symptoms as they feel now gives way to the sweet relief of a lessening in their intensity.

*Turn to Drop-It Practice when your reaction
to your symptoms is becoming more and
more mentally distressing.*

Sometimes a simple thought, such as "My symptoms aren't so good today," triggers a series of increasingly irrational thoughts until you're suddenly telling yourself alarming stories that go something like this: "These symptoms will take over the rest of my life; I'll never enjoy anything again."

When you realize this is happening, gently but firmly say to yourself *drop it*, and then turn your attention to some sensory experience—a sight, a sound, the physical sensation of your in- and out-breaths.

Drop-It Practice offers relief from stressful thought patterns because you cannot be lost in your stories if you're truly paying attention to what's happening in your immediate experience. If the stories start up again, try repeating the practice.

*Cultivate self-compassion to ease the mental
suffering that's accompanying your symptoms.*

Start with these words from Kahlil Gibran:
"Tenderness and kindness are not signs of
weakness and despair, but manifestations of
strength and resolution." Resolve to do whatever you can to treat yourself kindly.

Self-compassion includes taking care of
your daily needs, doing some things you
enjoy, and speaking kindly to yourself by
finding words that articulate how hard it is
to cope with your symptoms. Once you have
your words, repeat them gently to yourself.
They might be "I'm frustrated that I have the
same symptoms day after day" or even "I'm
sorry you're sick, sweet body, working so
hard to support me."

Expressing compassion for yourself in this
way lets you know that you care about your
suffering. This alone makes the severity of
your symptoms easier to bear.

*Cultivate equanimity to ease the mental
suffering that's present due your aversion
toward your symptoms.*

Equanimity is an even-tempered peace of mind
that arises when you feel okay about your life
as it is instead of being stuck in endless longing
for it to be different.

Consider these words from the Thai Forest
monk Ajahn Chah:

> If you let go a little, you will
> have a little peace. If you let
> go a lot, you will have a lot of
> peace. If you let go completely,
> you will have complete peace
> and freedom. Your struggles
> with the world will have come
> to an end.

Surrendering to how your symptoms feel at the moment is a tall order, but clinging to the way you wish they'd feel only adds mental suffering to the mix.

Try letting go of your aversion to your symptoms. Do it one small step at a time, as Ajahn Chah suggests.

*Describe your symptoms in a neutral way,
leaving out emotionally charged adjectives
and self-referential terms.*

Compare these two ways of describing pain: "I'm in unbearable pain" versus "Pain is present."

When you omit the adjective "unbearable" from your description of pain (as in the second example), you're acknowledging the pain, but you're not adding an emotional charge. And when you omit the self-referential term "I'm," you're still saying that pain is present, but you're treating it as due to causes and conditions, not as something personal.

Try this approach with any symptom—physical or mental. For instance: "Deep fatigue is present" or "Anxiety is happening." Describing symptoms in this neutral way can even keep them from intensifying.

Listen to your body, and pace yourself.

In my experience, this is the best way to get symptoms to calm down. Start by listening to your body. If it's telling you to stop visiting, bring that visit to a close as soon as possible. If it's telling you to lie down, find a way to lie down. Before I became ill, I hardly ever listened to my body. Now it has my ear all the time.

Pacing takes many forms: you can make a schedule for the day that includes rest periods; you can set the intention to do tasks more slowly; you can decide what you *think* you can do on a given day and then only do 50 percent of it.

Of course, sometimes the best of pacing plans must give way to unexpected events of the day. That's okay. Simply make plans to pace yourself the next day, or, if that's not possible, the next.

Look for something pleasing to distract you
from focusing solely on your symptoms.

It's not unusual for the chronically ill to turn their attention inward and focus on their symptoms. Of course, doing this for the purpose of self-care is a good idea. But focusing solely on symptoms can also give rise to painful emotions, such as frustration, anger, and even fear.

An enjoyable distraction can ease your mental suffering. Create one yourself, perhaps by putting on some music. Or, shift your attention from your symptoms to the world around you. Maybe you'll see a flower, blowing in the wind . . .

Today, alone,
I distract myself with flowers
that attract my eyes like magnets.

The wind roughhouses,
bending them over.
—the eleventh-century poet Ibn
   Zydun

*In whatever way you're able, reach out to
another person.*

Reaching out to others who could use your
encouragement and support carries a triple
benefit: it helps them; it takes your mind off
your symptoms; and it's good for your emotional health.

Showing that you care about another person can take the simplest form—a thoughtful
card sent through the mail, a texted "Hello,
how are you?"

The smallest gesture of kindness on your
part could easily be the highlight of someone
else's day. It's also likely to make your symptoms easier to bear because you're focusing
on another person instead of on yourself.

*Accept the possibility that chronic illness,
along with its symptoms, may be with you
the rest of your life.*

You have to decide if this perspective would be beneficial for you. Personally, the day I accepted the possibility that this might be true for me, to my surprise, instead of feeling sad and disheartened, I was relieved, as if a heavy burden had been lifted—the burden to regain my health at all costs.

It doesn't mean you should stop looking for new treatments (I'm still looking), but you might benefit, as I have, from accepting the possibility that chronic illness may be a permanent part your life journey.

Without carrying the burden of feeling that you must regain your health at any cost (financial or emotional), you can dedicate yourself to making the best life you can, chronic illness included.

THE CHALLENGE
Handling the Emotional Pain of Receiving Cursory or Dismissive Medical Care

If this has happened to you (it has to me more than once), you know it feels terrible. Sometimes I've been bewildered: "Why isn't this doctor paying attention to what I'm saying?" Other times, it's felt like an emotional gut punch.

And yet, despite the disappointment, frustration, and even anger that follows on the heels of an encounter like this, all of us have to move on.

Let these words from Maya Angelou serve as inspiration: "You may not control all the events that happen to you, but you can decide not to be reduced by them."

Here are some suggestions and practices to keep you from being "reduced" by what happened. I suggest you start by considering what's on the next page . . .

*Ask yourself "Am I sure?" before deciding
that your initial assessment of this medical
encounter was accurate.*

The Vietnamese Zen master Thich Nhat Hanh
suggests asking yourself "Am I sure?" before
deciding that your initial reaction to an interaction accurately reflected what went on. Are
you sure the person you saw didn't want to
help you? Maybe he or she had an overwhelming workload that day.

In this way, asking "Am I sure?" keeps you
from believing distressing thoughts before
you've even considered if they're a valid expla-
nation of what happened: "That doctor didn't
want to have anything to do with me." Are you
sure? If you're not, and if you've received good
medical care from this person in the past, it
might be smart to try one more appointment.

If you *do* decide that you were treated
poorly, try what follows on the next few pages.

Try Drop-It Practice if you're trapped in a round of increasingly stressful thoughts about the appointment.

When you're disappointed about something, a seemingly neutral thought, such as "That appointment didn't go as planned," can set off a series of increasingly stressful reactions until you're suddenly lost in irrational stories that go something like this: "It's absolutely clear—I'm not worth any doctor's time or effort."

When you realize this is happening, gently but firmly say to yourself *drop it*, and then turn your attention to some sensory experience—a sight, a sound, the physical sensation of your in- and out-breaths.

Drop-It Practice cuts off painful thought patterns by redirecting your attention to what's going on in your immediate experience. If you start to get lost in your stories again, try repeating the practice.

Turn to Three-Breath Practice to shift your attention from the appointment to what's going on in your field of awareness right now.

Pause and bring your full attention to the physical sensation of three consecutive in-breaths and out-breaths. Take your time.

Because the sensations of the breath always take place in the present moment, this practice *puts* you in the present moment. This not only breaks the hold of stressful thoughts and emotions related to the appointment, it also offers the opportunity for you to find something pleasant and enjoyable that's going on in your field of awareness right now.

Three-Breath and Drop-It Practices work well together. They both train you to bring your attention to what's present in your experience right now instead of being trapped in a cycle of increasingly stressful thoughts and emotions.

Let self-compassion be a healing balm for any frustration or anger that's lingering after the appointment.

Treating yourself with compassion, both in your speech and your actions, will ease your emotional pain. Compassionate action includes taking good care of your body and making sure you do some things that are fulfilling or just plain fun.

To speak compassionately to yourself, think of words that express how painful it was to have been treated poorly. Then gently repeat them to yourself with as much kindness as you can muster. Your words might be "Having been treated that way really hurt" or "I feel both angry and sad that I wasn't taken seriously."

When you give voice to your feelings in this way, you're showing yourself that you care about your suffering. This alone will ease your emotional pain and make what happened easier to bear.

*Cultivate equanimity to help overcome the
mental suffering that's arisen due to this
disheartening interaction.*

From the Tibetan teacher Lama Yeshe: "If you
expect your life to be up and down, your mind
will be much more peaceful." The peacefulness
of equanimity arises when you truly see that
sometimes life goes your way, and sometimes
it doesn't.

Draw inspiration from the Thai Forest
monk Ajahn Jumnian who, with joyful serenity, told a group of us that he felt okay about
his life no matter what happened. Faced with
this challenge, he'd have said something like
"If the appointment had gone well, that
would have been nice, but it's okay that it
didn't. Some doctors come through for you
and some don't. I'll keep looking."

The evenness of temper and peace of mind
that characterize equanimity make it well
worth your effort to cultivate.

*Don't give up your search for
decent medical care.*

Heed this advice from the ancient Chinese sage Lao Tzu: "Respond intelligently even to unintelligent treatment." The intelligent response to receiving cursory or dismissive treatment would *not* be: "That doctor didn't want to treat me. I give up." Unfortunately, self-blame tends to follow on the heels of giving up, and that can keep you from taking constructive action, such as looking for another doctor.

By contrast, evoking compassion for yourself over what happened is an intelligent response. You're letting yourself know that you understand how disappointing and hard this has been. Feeling understood paves the way for you to take action to seek better medical care.

To echo those words of Maya Angelou, you're making sure you haven't been "reduced" by what happened.

THE CHALLENGE
Coping Skillfully with Disappointment and Sadness When a New Treatment Didn't Help

It's natural to get your hopes up when you try a new treatment. I always do. Then, of course, it's terribly disappointing if it doesn't work out.

Allowing that disappointment to escalate into full-blown anger, however, only makes you feel worse physically and emotionally. Bottom line: sometimes a treatment helps; sometimes it doesn't.

Take extra good care of yourself while you come to terms with what happened. The suggestions and practices that follow will help you through this tough period.

*Recognize that your emotional reaction
to the outcome of this treatment is as
changeable as the weather.*

Even though what happened with this treatment has left you feeling sad—even distraught—emotions, like the weather, are in constant flux. They don't stay the same for long.

Be patient with yourself while you wait out these painful emotions, just like you'd wait for a storm to pass. Patience and compassion for your suffering help you stay open to the possibility that the next treatment will be helpful.

*Keep a Don't-Know Mind about future
treatments.*

When it comes to future treatments, you don't
know if the next one will help or if it will be
disappointing. You don't know because you
don't know the future. No one does.

The Korean Zen master Seung Sahn's
instruction to keep a Don't-Know Mind is
an invitation to lay down the burden of constantly striving to know the unknowable.

Keeping a Don't-Know Mind is also
invaluable as a technique for preventing you
from believing upsetting thoughts, such as
"No treatment is ever going to work for me."
You can't possibly know if this is true. Stay
open to the possibility that the next treatment
will be helpful.

Turn to self-compassion to alleviate any emotional pain you're experiencing as a result of the treatment not having worked.

When you treat yourself with compassion, you open the door to healing yourself emotionally. Self-compassion includes speaking kindly to yourself and taking compassionate action on your behalf.

To engage in compassionate speech, find words that articulate how hard it is to cope with a treatment that didn't work. Then recite them to yourself in a gentle and soothing manner, words such as "It's frustrating to be let down by yet another treatment" or "It's a struggle to accept what happened without bitterness."

When you speak to yourself with understanding in this way, you're letting yourself know that you care about your suffering. This alone will ease your emotional pain.

*Use Three-Breath Practice to shift your
attention from the treatment to what's going
on in your field of awareness right now.*

If you're struck in troubling thoughts and
emotions related to this treatment, *pause,* and
shift your attention to the physical sensation
of three consecutive in- and out-breaths. This
practice prevents you from remaining lost
in painful thoughts and emotions because
it grounds you in the present moment—
specifically in the physical sensations that
accompany your breathing.

Every time you engage in Three-Breath
Practice you're easing your emotional pain,
because you're bringing your attention to
what's present in your experience right now
instead of agonizing over a treatment that
didn't work.

Turn to Three-Breath Practice for relief at
any time and in any place.

Cultivate equanimity to ease the mental suffering that's stemming from this treatment not having worked.

Equanimity is an even-tempered peace of mind that arises when you're able to graciously accept that sometimes life goes well for you and sometimes it's terribly disappointing. Taoism refers to this as the ten thousand joys and the ten thousand sorrows.

Draw inspiration from the Thai Forest monk Ajahn Jumnian who, with joyful serenity, told a group of us that he felt okay about his life no matter how it unfolded. Faced with this challenge, he'd have said something like "If this treatment had helped, that would have been nice, but it's okay that it didn't. It just wasn't right for me. Let me figure out what to do next."

The evenness of temper and calm acceptance that characterize equanimity make it well worth your effort to cultivate.

*Work on giving in to what happened
instead of giving up.*

Be careful not to let the calm acceptance of equanimity turn into indifference or resignation, as in "That treatment didn't work, but who cares? I give up." Self-blame tends to follow on the heels of giving up. This can prevent you from taking constructive action to help yourself, such as continuing to stay informed about new treatment options.

By contrast, *giving in* brings with it a sense of relief—a sweet surrender to what you cannot change at this moment, while remaining committed to doing what you can to ease both your physical and mental suffering.

THE CHALLENGE
Responding with Patience and Courage to the Appearance of a New Medical Problem

The sudden appearance of a new medical problem on top of your existing health struggles is a potent reminder that life isn't necessarily fair. In my experience, constantly trying to make it fair is an oppressive burden.

Casting aside this burden leaves you free to turn your attention to taking good care of your body and to easing the mental suffering that's accompanying this new illness or injury.

Here are some recommendations and practices for helping you to accept your life as it is, even when it takes an unwelcome turn.

Ask yourself "Am I sure?" before concluding that you won't be able to cope with this new medical problem.

The Zen master Thich Nhat Hanh suggests asking yourself "Am I sure?" before deciding that your immediate reaction to something that happened is an accurate assessment of what you can expect in the future.

In this way, asking "Am I sure?" keeps you from believing alarming thoughts before you've even considered if they're a rational prediction of what's going to happen: "This new diagnosis will make my chronic illness impossible to live with." You don't know if this is true.

Rather than jumping to worst-case-scenario conclusions, ask "Am I sure?" Then you can take a wait-and-see attitude, which will ease your anxiety about the impact of the new diagnosis.

*Turn to Three-Breath Practice to help
alleviate any worry or even fear you're
experiencing as a result of learning about
this new medical problem.*

When you become aware that you're lost in disturbing thoughts and emotions relating to this new medical problem, *pause*, and switch your attention to the physical sensation of three in- and three out-breaths in a row. Take your time.

Three-Breath Practice grounds you in the present moment because that's where the sensations of the breath always take place. Bringing your attention to the breath in this way offers relief from troubling thoughts and emotions related to this new medical problem. It also provides the opportunity for you to find something pleasant and enjoyable going on in your field of awareness right now.

Three-Breath Practice can be done at any time and any place. Repeat as necessary!

*When thoughts about this new medical
problem give rise to frustration, anger, or
even fear, turn to self-compassion.*

Self-compassion asks only that you be kind to
yourself, both in your speech and your actions.
Compassionate action includes taking care of
your needs and making sure you do some special things for yourself.

To speak compassionately to yourself,
think of words that capture the emotional
pain of being diagnosed with a new condition. Then repeat them to yourself in a soothing manner. Your words might be similar to
these: "It's so hard to have this injury on top
of my ongoing illness" or "I'm worried and
even scared about my ability to cope with this
new diagnosis."

Expressing compassion for yourself in this
way lets you know that you care about your
suffering. This alone will make this new medical problem easier to adjust to.

Cultivate equanimity to ease the mental suffering that's been triggered by the discovery of a new medical problem.

Equanimity is a feeling of even-tempered serenity that arises when you're able to accept your life as it is without aversion or bitterness, instead of being stuck in continuous longing for it to be different.

A student once asked the spiritual teacher Jiddu Krishnamurti what his secret to peace and contentment was. He leaned over and whispered to the student: "I don't mind what happens."

To cultivate equanimity in this way, start by gently acknowledging any worry or fear that's present due to learning about this new medical problem. Then try to imagine what it would be like to not mind that this has happened.

This can be a challenge, so if it was too hard to imagine, wait a bit and try again.

*Recognize that the best medical course of
action may not always be clear.*

If you're like me, you didn't realize until you
became chronically ill how many gray areas
still exist in medicine. If you got a bacterial
infection, you took an antibiotic. If you got a
viral infection, you waited it out with the help
of over-the-counter medications.

But once you entered the world of chronic
pain and illness, you probably discovered
what I did: it's not always clear what treatments to try.

The best you can do is gather all the information you can, and then make a treatment
decision based on what appears to be the
wisest choice in your circumstances. Then
acknowledge with compassion for yourself
that the outcome of the treatment is going to
be uncertain.

THE CHALLENGE
Accepting without Bitterness How Restricted Your Life Has Become, Socially and Otherwise

I still get sad when I think of everything I've missed out on due to chronic illness. Particularly hard for me has been my inability to take part in family gatherings.

Chronic illness can significantly alter your ability to socialize and to engage in activities you used to love. It's a challenge to adjust to this change.

When my limitations get me down, I turn for help to the ideas and practices on the next few pages. May they be of benefit to you, too.

*Take comfort in knowing that you're okay
even though your limitations are a source of
emotional suffering at the moment.*

Let these words from the Zen teacher Charlotte Joko Beck reassure you that you're okay: "Our life is always all right. There's nothing wrong with it. Even if we have horrendous problems, it's just our life."

Because there's nothing wrong with your life, *there's nothing wrong with you.* Yes, you're unhappy right now about how restricted your life has become, but it's okay to feel that way. As Joko Beck said, it's just your life—in this case, your life with chronic illness.

Recognize that constant change and the lack of control it implies come with being human.

Life is one surprise after another. Some of them will be to your liking; some will not. If you could control what happened to you, you wouldn't impose limitations on yourself. But life doesn't work that way. At some point, all of us face health challenges that affect our ability to continue taking part in activities we love.

Because you have little control over what changes are in store for you in the future, it would be wise to make a commitment to appreciate the people and the activities that you're able to enjoy right now.

Work with Drop-It Practice when your reaction to your limitations is becoming increasingly upsetting.

When you're thinking about how restricted your life has become, a simple inquiry, such as "I wonder how long I'll be able to socialize today," can mushroom into a series of increasingly irrational thoughts until you're telling yourself alarming stories that go something like this: "I'll never have fun again."

When this happens, gently but firmly say to yourself *drop it*, and then turn your attention to some sensory experience—a sight, a sound, the physical sensation of your in- and out-breaths.

Drop-It Practice cuts off painful thought patterns by redirecting your attention to what's going on in your immediate experience. It also helps you find things to enjoy that are available to you right now, despite your limitations.

*Think of words that articulate how hard it
is to be so limited in what you can do, and
repeat them gently to yourself.*

Spend a few minutes finding just the right
words—words that reflect how difficult it is to
cope with your limitations. Then bring them to
mind and repeat them soothingly to yourself.
Your words might be some version of these:
"I wish with all my heart that I could join the
family for dinner" or "I'm sad and even a bit
resentful that I can't go my friend's party."

When you give voice to your feelings in
this manner, you're letting yourself know that
you care about your suffering. This alone will
ease your mental suffering and make your
limitations easier to live with.

Let the kindness of self-compassion ease any frustration, resentment, or anger you're feeling due to being so restricted in what you can do.

From the 14th Dalai Lama: "My religion is very simple. My religion is kindness." Use his words as inspiration to treat yourself with compassion as you adjust to this drastic change in your life.

Being kind to yourself loosens the grip of painful emotions, and this frees you to look for possibilities you may not have considered—things you can do that are both enjoyable and within your limitations. This is compassion in action.

As your ability to cultivate self-compassion grows, it will become easier to take on the challenging task of learning how to live a rich and fulfilling life despite your limitations.

Cultivate equanimity to relieve the mental suffering that's stemming from feeling so limited in what you can do.

Start with these words from the ancient Greek philosopher Epictetus: "Make the best use of what is in your power and take the rest as it happens."

This quotation captures the essence of equanimity—that evenness of temper and sense of well-being that arise when you're able to accept your limitations without bitterness.

"Take the rest as it happens" doesn't imply indifference or resignation. It challenges you to embrace your life as it is, limitations included.

*Don't glorify the past by fooling yourself
into thinking that you had no limitations
before becoming chronically ill.*

In the words of Marcel Proust, "Remembrance of things past is not necessarily the remembrance of things as they were." Be careful not to look upon your life before chronic illness as always carefree and unlimited. It wasn't. You couldn't do whatever you wanted, whenever you wanted. No one can.

It's fun to enjoy fond memories of the past, but that's not the same as fooling yourself into thinking that you were always untroubled and happy back then. Like everyone else, you had your share of frustrations and disappointments. Life is a mixture of joys and sorrows for everyone.

Be a friend to yourself by being realistic about what your life was like before chronic illness!

*Practice feeling joy for those who have an
active social life and are able to engage in
activities they love.*

Consider these words from Lama Zopa Rin-
poche: "Always practice rejoicing for others—
whether your friend or your enemy. If you
cannot practice rejoicing, no matter how long
you live, you will not be happy."

Feeling joy for others is a potent antidote for envy and resentment—two sources
of emotional suffering that so easily arise
when you start comparing your life to that
of others.

Every time you generate a bit of joy for
others, you're planting a seed that you can
cultivate. As you become more skilled at this,
something special can happen—you may
feel such a strong connection to those you're
cultivating joy for that you'll suddenly find
yourself feeling joyful, too, as if you're taking
part in what they're doing.

*If your health allows, consider going outside
your limitations when there's something
special you want to do.*

Some people have to stay strictly within the restrictions imposed by their chronic illness. Others don't, even though doing more than they can easily handle can lead to a flare in symptoms.

If you have the flexibility to go beyond your limitations and an activity or event is special to you, for your emotional well-being, it may be worth the "payback." You have to decide what's best for you.

On occasion, I've gone beyond my limitations by attending a special event, such as a wedding. I've never regretted it. That said, if this type of event is not close to home, I can't go. It's essential to pay attention to just how far you can stretch your limitations. Having done that, hopefully, sometimes you can participate in something that's special to you.

THE CHALLENGE
Easing the Heartache of Feeling Disregarded or Even Not Believed by Family and Friends

Most people don't realize that someone can look fine but be chronically ill, physically or mentally. Unless a chronic illness is visible (and it usually isn't), family and friends may discount or even not believe that you're sick or in pain. This misconception can persist even after you've explained your condition. It's hurtful and demoralizing.

You've probably had to endure this dreaded comment more than once: "But you don't *look* sick." One reason for this is that, if you're like me, you usually have to use adrenaline to get through extended interactions. Unfortunately, it can take days for your body to recover from this.

I hope what follows will ease any anger or other mental suffering that's resulting from feeling disregarded or not believed by those you care about the most.

Start by asking yourself "Am I sure?"
before deciding that family and friends are
callously disregarding you.

The Zen master Thich Nhat Hanh suggests that
you ask yourself "Am I sure?" before deciding
that your assessment of someone is correct.
You can set yourself up for needless heartache
if you erroneously jump to the conclusion that
a friend or family member is callously disregarding you. There are several reasons why
some of the people you care about the most
might not be a source of support for you right
now.

First, like many other people, they may be
woefully uneducated about chronic illness
and not know that someone can look fine but
feel terrible. As a result, they may not realize
how sick or in pain you truly are.

Second, they may care deeply about you
but be facing difficulties of their own, such as

family, work, or even health problems. The next page offers a third reason why loved ones may not be a source of support.

Lack of support from family and friends may not be about you but, instead, be a sign of their own anxiety and fear about chronic illness.

Sometimes people do believe that you're chronically ill but still can't lend support because they're uncomfortable around others who are struggling with their health. Our culture does a poor job of preparing us for the fact that everyone will face pain or illness at some point in life and, when it happens, be in need of extra support and kindness.

Loved ones who don't stay in touch may think about you frequently and wish you well, but not be a part of your life due to their own anxiety and fear about pain and illness. If this is the case, there's no reason to take their absence personally: it's about them, not you. See if you can cultivate compassion for the anxiety and fear they're suffering over something that's natural to the human condition.

Turn to Drop-It Practice when you're caught in a web of painful thoughts and emotions about friends and family.

When you're worried about the state of your relationships, a seemingly simple thought, such as "I wish people understood my illness better," can trigger a series of increasingly irrational thoughts until you're suddenly lost in alarming stories that go something like this: "No one will ever believe how sick and in pain I am. I hate them all."

Hostility toward others only makes you feel worse, so if you realize you're engaging in this, gently but firmly say to yourself *drop it*. Then turn your attention to some sensory experience—a sight, a sound, the physical sensation of your in- and out-breaths.

By focusing your attention on what's happening in your immediate experience, Drop-It Practice offers relief from painful thoughts and emotions about others.

Let self-compassion ease any anger or other mental suffering you're experiencing as a result of how others are treating you.

Self-compassion includes taking action to ease your suffering (such as doing something nice for yourself) and speaking kindly to yourself by finding words that articulate the emotional pain of feeling disregarded or disbelieved by others. Once you have your words, repeat them gently to yourself. They might be "I'm so hurt that my friends don't ask how I'm doing" or "It breaks my heart that some family members don't believe that I'm in pain."

When you give voice to your feelings like this, you're letting yourself know that you care about your suffering. This alone will ease your emotional pain.

Finally, as you repeat your chosen words, try stroking one arm with the hand of the other in reassurance; this never fails to ease my mental suffering.

*Try educating family and friends about
what life is like for you.*

Unless you tell them, those you care about the
most may not understand what it's like for you
to live with chronic illness.

If you're able to use a computer (not everyone can), email is an effective and nonstressful
way to communicate with others. Take as long
as you want to compose and edit what you've
written until you're satisfied that it conveys
exactly what you want to share. I suggest that
you be descriptive and avoid complaining (the
latter can be a challenge at times!).

You might include how unpredictable your
symptoms are from day to day, and explain
that this is why making plans is so problematic. This type of information can significantly improve a relationship. If your attempt
to explain what your life is like doesn't have
the desired effect, at least you gave it your
best shot.

*Cultivate equanimity to help you let go of
any bitterness or anger you're feeling toward
family and friends.*

Equanimity arises when you can accept without bitterness or anger that some loved ones may not come through for you.

Consider these words from the Thai Forest monk Ajahn Chah:

> If you let go a little, you will
> have a little peace. If you let
> go a lot, you will have a lot of
> peace. If you let go completely,
> you will have complete peace
> and freedom. Your struggles
> with the world will have come
> to an end.

Try letting go of your aversion to those who've let you down. Do it one small step at a time, as Ajahn Chah suggests.

Clinging to the way you want others to be only adds mental suffering to the mix. It's better to stick with family and friends who support you and, if possible, let the others slip out of your life.

Think about other people you could reach out
to, either in person or in cyberspace.

If you're able to use a computer, online chronic illness groups can be a rich source of support, although you may have to hunt around a bit until you find people whose perspective on illness—and life in general— resonates with you.

When you find others who understand from firsthand experience what your life is like, it feels as if you've been thrown a lifeline. Suddenly, you're being heard and supported and understood.

Also consider getting in touch with an old friend. Perhaps he or she has developed health problems, too, and you'll immediately realize that the two of you have a lot in common. A discovery like this can rekindle an old friendship fast.

THE CHALLENGE
Alleviating the Pain of Loneliness

The dramatic change in lifestyle that usually accompanies chronic illness can lead to painful feelings of loneliness. Previously, you may have been in the company of others every day; suddenly, you're by yourself most of the time.

I find it helpful to distinguish between *being alone* and *feeling lonely*.

Being alone, in itself, is a neutral state, neither positive nor negative. The philosopher and theologian Paul Tillich said this about being alone: "Language . . . has created the word 'loneliness' to express the pain of being alone. And it has created the word 'solitude' to express the glory of being alone."

May what follows help you take the first steps toward turning the pain of loneliness into the glory of solitude.

Take comfort in knowing you are not alone
in your loneliness.

Millions of people understand how you feel.
Roy Orbison expressed it this way: "Only the
lonely know the way I feel tonight."

Bringing to mind others who are lonely
and evoking compassion for them and for
yourself over your shared circumstances can
make you feel deeply connected to them. This
can ease your own loneliness.

*Think of words that capture the pain of
loneliness, and repeat them to yourself in a
gentle and soothing manner.*

Here's an example attributed to the Talmud:
"The highest form of wisdom is kindness."
Find those kind words—ones that resonate
with you personally—and bring them to mind
with a gentle and soothing voice. Your words
might be similar to these: "It's dispiriting to
feel so lonely" or "I'm incredibly sad that I'm
not with my friends tonight."

Expressing compassion for yourself in
this way lets you know that you care about
your suffering. This makes loneliness easier
to bear, and also makes it easier to patiently
wait for it to pass out of your mind.

If you find yourself focusing on loneliness, examine whether it's for a constructive purpose or whether it's only making you feel worse.

When you're feeling lonely, there's a tendency to focus on it exclusively. This is beneficial if your intention is to shed light on what gives rise to loneliness. For instance, if you know that it's triggered by certain interactions or activities on your part, you can try to avoid them.

However, if your focus is on how bad loneliness feels, this can increase its intensity. If this is what you're doing, a pleasing distraction can help by shifting your attention from loneliness to what the world around you has to offer right at this moment. You could put on some music or go outside for a while. Come up with what you think would be enjoyable to do and then *do it*, even if you have to apply what I call "gentle force" to get yourself going. This is self-compassion in action.

Use Three-Breath Practice to shift your attention from feeling lonely to what's going on in your field of experience right now.

When loneliness feels overwhelming, *pause*, and bring your full attention to the physical sensation of three consecutive in-breaths and out-breaths. This simple but powerful practice loosens the grip of loneliness because it shifts your attention to what's going on in your immediate experience—specifically to the physical sensations that accompany breathing.

After taking those three in- and out-breaths, you can simply enjoy the relief of having relaxed into the present moment, or you can look for a pleasant distraction as discussed in the previous suggestion.

Three-Breath Practice opens your heart and mind to the possibility that enjoyable experiences are within your reach right now. Return to this practice often.

*See if you can make friends with loneliness
by letting it keep you company.*

This suggestion was inspired by a passage in an Ann Packer novel: "Loneliness is a funny thing. It's almost like another person. After a while it will keep you company if you let it."

Let it keep you company by calmly giving in to loneliness instead of giving up in anger. Giving up takes this form: "I hate this feeling of loneliness. I want to get rid of it, but I can't. I give up." This kind of thinking makes you feel like a failure and leaves you just as lonely, if not lonelier.

By contrast, gently giving in to loneliness arouses self-compassion because, when you treat loneliness with kindness and understanding, you're treating yourself with kindness and understanding. In this way, you're befriending this difficult emotion.

*Each evening, write down something fun or
fulfilling that you plan to do the next day.*

Putting your plan in writing increases the
likelihood that you'll follow through with it
because you've made it part of your schedule
for the next day.

Of course, sometimes unexpected things
come up and you can't keep to your plan.
When this happens, tell yourself, "That's life!
No blame!" And then, that evening, write
down something fun or fulfilling that you
plan to do the next day.

Recognize that feelings of loneliness are as changeable as the weather.

You may feel as if you'll always be lonely, but emotions are in constant flux, arising and passing, just like weather patterns. In the words of the poet Rainer Maria Rilke: "No feeling is final."

Without trying to force any sadness to go away, be patient with your loneliness. It's likely that by tomorrow, it will have eased a bit—and perhaps the next day, a bit more.

And the day after that, it might even turn into Paul Tillich's glorious solitude . . .

THE CHALLENGE
Managing Caregiver Burnout Wisely

Dear Caregivers,

You are my heroes. Many of you are invisible to others as you quietly and unobtrusively fulfill your responsibilities to the person in your care, often while holding down another job.

It's likely you were thrust into this role without any training and maybe even without notice. Please remember that it's not your job to fix the person in your care, nor are you responsible for his or her happiness. Neither of these are within your power.

Take good care of yourselves. To ease your burden and help with burnout, try what follows on the next few pages.

Recognize that impermanence and the lack of control it implies come with the human condition.

John Lennon said it this way: "Life is what happens to you when you're busy making other plans." If you could control the course your life was going to take, you probably wouldn't have included plans to be a caregiver. Yet it's not uncommon for people to suddenly find themselves in this role and feel completely unprepared for it, so you are not alone. Just knowing that can help ease the mental suffering of burnout.

In addition, the impermanent nature of life can help you cope with feeling burned out by encouraging you to find activities that both you and the person in your care can enjoy right now.

Take solace in knowing that you're okay
even though you're feeling burned out at the
moment.

Let these words from the Zen teacher Charlotte Joko Beck reassure you that you're okay: "Our life is always all right. There's nothing wrong with it. Even if we have horrendous problems, it's just our life."

Because there's nothing wrong with your life, *there's nothing wrong with you.* Yes, you're feeling burned out right now, but it's okay to feel that way. As Joko Beck said, it's just your life—in this case, your life as a caregiver.

*Work with Drop-It Practice when you're
stuck in a cycle of increasingly stressful
thoughts regarding your role as caregiver.*

When you're feeling burned out, an otherwise unremarkable thought, such as "I have several things to take care of today," can set off a series of increasingly irrational thoughts until you're suddenly telling yourself depressing stories that go something like this: "I'll never get time to myself. All my life plans are ruined."

When you realize this is happening, gently but firmly say to yourself *drop it*, and then turn your attention to some sensory experience—a sight, a sound, the physical sensation of your in- and out-breaths.

Drop-It Practice offers relief from stressful thought patterns because you cannot be lost in your stories if you're truly paying attention to what's happening in your immediate experience.

*Cultivate self-compassion to ease the mental
suffering that accompanies feeling burned out.*

Self-compassion is a source of deep comfort.
All you need to do is be kind to yourself, both
in your speech and your actions. Compassionate action can be as simple as doing something
special for yourself alone.

To engage in compassionate speech, find
words that directly express how hard it is to
feel burned out. Then recite them to yourself
as kindly and gently as you can, words such
as "It's a struggle to accept such a drastic
change in my life plans" or even "Sometimes
I resent having to be 'on duty' all the time."

When you give voice to your feelings like
this, you're showing yourself that you care
about your suffering. This will ease the emotional pain that accompanies burnout.

*Cultivate equanimity to help you through
this difficult period.*

Consider these words from Joseph Campbell: "We must let go of the life we have planned so as to accept the one that is waiting for us." Equanimity is a feeling of peace and contentment that arise when you're able to accept without bitterness that life doesn't always go as planned.

Draw inspiration from the Thai Forest monk Ajahn Jumnian who, with joyful serenity, told a group of us that he felt okay about his life no matter what happened. Faced with this challenge, he'd have said something like "It would be nice if I didn't have to be a caregiver, but it's okay. Life always takes unexpected turns. I'll make the best of this role and look for joy wherever I can find it."

The evenness of temper and peace of mind that characterize equanimity make it well worth your effort to cultivate.

Whenever possible, find time for yourself.

Work on carving out periods of time to pursue your own interests or to do something for yourself that's just plain fun. This may require careful planning but, along with finding others who can help you with your responsibilities, setting aside time for yourself is the best way to prevent caregiver burnout.

Don't be thrown off course if something unexpected comes up that makes it impossible to carry out your plans for a particular day. If this happens, accept it as an inevitable part of life, and start planning again for some time when you can be on your own.

*Keep a Don't-Know Mind about the health
of the person in your care.*

You don't know the extent to which your caregiver duties will stay the same or will change. You don't know because you don't know what the future has in store. No one does.

It's surprisingly liberating to be able to say, "I don't know." Those words free you to let your caregiver duties take what course they may without the futile effort on your part to control everything.

Keeping a Don't-Know Mind is also an invaluable way to stop yourself from believing distressing assumptions, such as "The future holds only misery for us." You can't know this, so stay open to the possibility that the condition of the person in your care will improve.

Final Thoughts

If you can change your mind,
you can change your life.
—WILLIAM JAMES

The more you work with the suggestions and practices in this book, the easier it will be to call them to mind when you're facing one of chronic illness's many challenges.

Also remember that, despite your best intentions, sometimes things fall apart and nothing goes as planned. When this happens, don't blame yourself. Keep what the Korean Zen master Ko Bong called a "Try Mind," and what I call a "Forgiving Mind": "I tried to respond with equanimity to what happened today, but I just couldn't. It's okay. I'll try again tomorrow."

My heartfelt wish for all of you is that you find a measure of peace and joy in the midst of the challenges you face. I'm confident that you can.

About the Author

Toni Bernhard is the author of the award-winning *How to Be Sick: A Buddhist-Inspired Guide for the Chronically Ill and Their Caregivers*; *How to Live Well with Chronic Pain and Illness*; and *How to Wake Up: A Buddhist-Inspired Guide to Navigating Joy and Sorrow*. Until forced to retire due to illness, Toni was a law professor at the University of California–Davis, serving six years as the dean of students. She has been a practicing Buddhist for over twenty-five years. Her popular blog, *Turning Straw into Gold*, is hosted by *Psychology Today* online. She can be found on the web at ToniBernhard.com.

What to Read Next
from Wisdom Publications

How to Be Sick: A Buddhist-Inspired Guide for the Chronically Ill and Their Caregivers
Toni Bernhard

Full of insights and practices hard-won from Toni's own ongoing life experience, this is a must-read for anyone who is—or who might one day be—sick.

How to Live Well with Chronic Pain and Illness: A Mindful Guide
Toni Bernhard

"Toni shows us the difference between pain and suffering, and shows us what it can mean for how we live: that our lives can still be joyful."
—David R. Loy, author of *A New Buddhist Path*

How to Wake Up: A Buddhist-Inspired Guide to Navigating Joy and Sorrow
Toni Bernhard

"This is a book for everyone."
—Alida Brill, author of *Dancing at the River's Edge*

A Heart Full of Peace
Joseph Goldstein

"In this short but substantive volume, Joseph Goldstein, who lectures and leads retreats around the world, presents his thoughts on the practice of compassion, love, kindness, restraint, a skillful mind, and a peaceful heart as an antidote to the materialism of our age."
—*Spirituality & Practice*

About Wisdom Publications

Wisdom Publications is the leading publisher of classic and contemporary Buddhist books and practical works on mindfulness. To learn more about us or to explore our other books, please visit our website at wisdomexperience,org or contact us at the address below.

Wisdom Publications
199 Elm Street
Somerville, MA 02144 USA

We are a 501(c)(3) organization, and donations in support of our mission are tax deductible.

Wisdom Publications is affiliated with the Foundation for the Preservation of the Mahayana Tradition (FPMT).